CW00588952

Get fit with a balanced Mediterranean Meal

Easy, low-calorie recipes for a healthier lifestyle

Lana Green

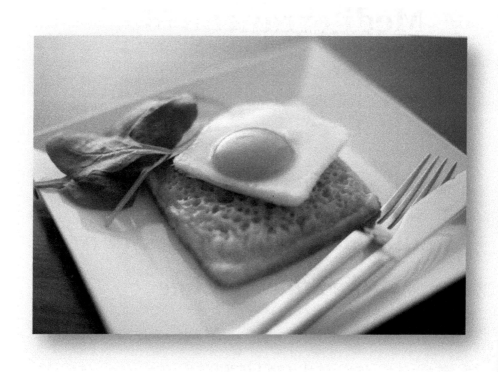

© **copyright 2021 – all rights reserved.**

the content contained within this book may not be reproduced, duplicated or transmitted without direct written permission from the author or the publisher.

under no circumstances will any blame or legal responsibility be held against the publisher, or author, for any damages, reparation, or monetary loss due to the information contained within this book. either directly or indirectly.

legal notice:

this book is copyright protected. this book is only for personal use. you cannot amend, distribute, sell, use, quote or paraphrase any part, or the content within this book, without the consent of the author or publisher.

disclaimer notice:

please note the information contained within this document is for educational and entertainment purposes only. all effort has been executed to present accurate, up to date, and reliable, complete information. no warranties of any kind are declared or implied. readers acknowledge that the author is not engaging in the rendering of legal, financial, medical or professional advice. the content within this book has been derived from various sources. please consult a licensed professional before attempting any techniques outlined in this book.

by reading this document, the reader agrees that under no circumstances is the author responsible for any losses, direct or indirect, which are incurred as a result of the use of information contained within this document, including, but not limited to, — errors, omissions, or inaccuracies.

Table of Contents

Bulgur Bowl

Prep Time: 10 min

Cook Time: 0 min

Serve: 4

Ingredients:

- 6 oz salmon, boiled, chopped

- ½ cup bulgur, cooked

- 1 cup fresh cilantro, chopped

- 1 cup tomato, chopped

- 3 tbsp. lemon juice

- 1 tbsp. olive oil

Preparation:

Put salmon, bulgur, cilantro, and tomato in the bowl. Add lemon juice and olive oil. Shake the mixture well and transfer in the serving bowls.

Boiled Bulgur with Kale

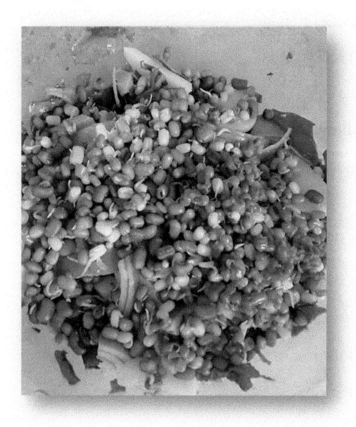

Prep Time: 10 min

Cook Time: 11 min

Serve: 6

Ingredients:

- 1 cup bulgur cups water

- 1 cup kale

- ½ zucchini, chopped

- ½ tsp. allspices

- 6 tbsp. olive oil

- 2 oz goat cheese, crumbled

Preparation:

1. Mix water and bulgur in the saucepan and cook boil for 11 minutes. Then cool the bulgur and mix it with chopped kale, zucchini, allspices, and olive oil.

2. Transfer the bulgur meal in the serving bowls and top with goat cheese.

Chicken and Rice Soup

Prep Time: 10 min

Cook Time: 20 min

Serve: 6

Ingredients:

- 4 cups chicken stock

- 1 cup of water

- 1-lb. chicken breast, shredded

- 1 cup of rice, cooked

- 3 egg yolks

- 3 tbsp. lemon juice

- 1/3 cup fresh parsley, chopped

- ½ tsp. salt

- ¼ tsp. ground black pepper

Preparation:

1. Pour water and chicken stock in the saucepan and bring to boil. Then pour one cup of the hot liquid in the food processor.

2. Add cooked rice, egg yolks, lemon juice, and salt. Blend the mixture until smooth. After this, transfer the smooth rice mixture into the saucepan with remaining chicken stock liquid.

3. Add shredded chicken breast, parsley, and ground black pepper. Boil the soup for 5 minutes more.

Tomato Bulgur

Prep Time: 5 min

Cook Time: 20 min

Serve: 3

Ingredients:

- ½ cup bulgur

- 1 onion, diced

- 3 tbsp. tomato paste

- ½ tsp. salt

- 2 tbsp. olive oil

- 1 cup of water

Preparation:

Melt the olive oil in the saucepan. Add diced onion and cook it until light brown. Then add bulgur and tomato paste. Stir the ingredients. Add water and cook the meal for 15 minutes.

Well spiced Lentil Soup with sour taste

Cook and Prep Time: 45 min

Serve: 6

Ingredients:

- water – 6 cups
- diced celery stalk - 1
- olive oil – 2 tbsps
- oregano sprig - 1
- chopped shallot – 1
- thyme sprig - 1
- chopped garlic clove – 1
- diced tomatoes – ½ cup
- cored and diced green bell pepper – 1
- sliced rhubarb stalks - 4
- cored and diced yellow bell pepper – 1
- green lentils – 1 cup
- diced carrot - 1
- vegetable stock – 2 cups

- Salt and pepper to taste

Preparation:

1. In a soup pot, heat the oil and stir in the garlic, bell peppers, shallots, carrot and celery. Soften it by cooking for 5 minutes and add stock, the lentils, water, rhubarb and water, also add tomatocs.

2. Add oregano sprig and thyme after seasoning with pepper and salt. For 20 minutes, cook on low heat. Best served chilled or warm.

Delicious and entertaining Lamb Veggie Soup

Cook and Prep Time: 1 ½ h

Serve: 8

Ingredients:

- water – 6 cups
- cubed pound lamb shoulder – 1 1 2
- lemon juice – 2 tbsps
- cauliflower florets – 2 cups
- olive oil – 2 tbsps
- basil sprig - 1
- chopped shallots – 2
- crushed tomatoes – 1 can
- diced carrots – 2
- thyme sprig - 1
- diced celery stalks – 2
- green peas – ½ cup
- grated ginger – ¼ tsp
- vegetable stock – 4 cups

- oregano sprig - 1

- Pepper and salt to taste

Preparation:

1. In a soup pot, heat the oil and stir in the lamb shoulder. Add stock and water after cooking on all sides for 5 minutes.

2. Add the remaining Ingredients: after cooking for 40 minutes and season with pepper and salt.

3. Cook it for another 20 minutes and serve the soup when it's still fresh.

Bulgur Mix

Prep Time: 10 min

Cook Time: 0 min

Serve: 3

Ingredients:

- ½ cup bulgur, cooked

- ¼ cup corn kernels, cooked

- ¼ cup chickpeas, cooked

- ¼ cup snap peas, cooked

- 4 tbsp. plain yogurt

Preparation:

Put all ingredients in the big bowl and carefully stir.

Aromatic Baked Brown Rice

Prep Time: 10 min

Cook Time: 20 min

Serve: 6

Ingredients:

- ½ cup minced fresh parsley

- ¾ cup jarred roasted

- red peppers, rinsed, patted dry, and chopped

- 1 cup chicken or vegetable broth

- 1½ cups long-grain brown rice, rinsed

- 2 onions, chopped fine

- 2¼ cups water

- 4 tsp. extra-virgin olive oil

- Grated Parmesan cheese

- Lemon wedges

- Salt and pepper

Preparation:

1. Place the oven rack in the centre of the oven and pre-heat your oven to 375°F. Heat oil in a Dutch oven on moderate heat until it starts to shimmer. Put in onions and 1 tsp. salt and cook, stirring intermittently, till they become tender and well browned, 12 to 14 minutes.

2. Mix in water and broth and bring to boil. Mix in rice, cover, and move pot to oven. Bake until rice becomes soft and liquid is absorbed, 65 to 70 minutes.

3. Remove pot from oven. Sprinkle red peppers over rice, cover, and allow to sit for about five minutes. Put in parsley to rice and fluff gently with fork to combine. Sprinkle with salt and pepper to taste. Serve with grated Parmesan and lemon wedges.

Aromatic Barley Pilaf

Prep Time: 10 min

Cook Time: 10 min

Serve: 6

Ingredients:

- ¼ cup minced fresh parsley

- 1 small onion, chopped fine

- 1½ cups pearl barley, rinsed

- 1½ tsp. lemon juice

- 1½ tsp. minced fresh thyme or ½ tsp. dried

- 2 garlic cloves, minced

- 2 tbsp. minced fresh chives

- 2½ cups water

- 3 tbsp. extra-virgin olive oil

- Salt and pepper

Preparation:

1. Heat oil in a big saucepan on moderate heat until it starts to shimmer. Put in onion and ½ tsp. salt and cook till they become tender, approximately five minutes. Mix in barley, garlic, and thyme and cook, stirring often, until barley is lightly toasted and aromatic, approximately three minutes.

2. Mix in water and bring to simmer. Decrease heat to low, cover, and simmer until barley becomes soft and water is absorbed, 20 to 40 minutes.

3. Remove from the heat, lay clean dish towel underneath lid and let pilaf sit for about ten minutes. Put in parsley, chives, and lemon juice to pilaf and fluff gently with fork to combine. Sprinkle with salt and pepper to taste. Serve.

Basmati Rice Pilaf Mix

Prep Time: 10 min

Cook Time: 15 min

Ingredients:

- ¼ cup currants

- ¼ cup sliced almonds, toasted

- ¼ tsp. ground cinnamon

- ½ tsp. ground turmeric

- 1 small onion, chopped fine

- 1 tbsp. extra-virgin olive oil

- 1½ cups basmati rice, rinsed

- 2 garlic cloves, minced

- 2¼ cups water

- Salt and pepper

Preparation:

1. Heat oil in a big saucepan on moderate heat until it starts to shimmer. Put in onion and ¼ tsp. salt and cook till they become tender, approximately five minutes. Put in rice, garlic, turmeric, and cinnamon and cook, stirring often, until grain edges begin to turn translucent, approximately three minutes.

2. Mix in water and bring to simmer. Decrease heat to low, cover, and simmer gently until rice becomes soft and water is absorbed, 16 to 18 minutes.

3. Remove from the heat, drizzle currants over pilaf. Cover, laying clean dish towel underneath lid, and let pilaf sit for about ten minutes. Put in almonds to pilaf and fluff gently with fork to combine. Sprinkle with salt and pepper to taste.

Brown Rice Salad with Asparagus, Goat Cheese, and Lemon

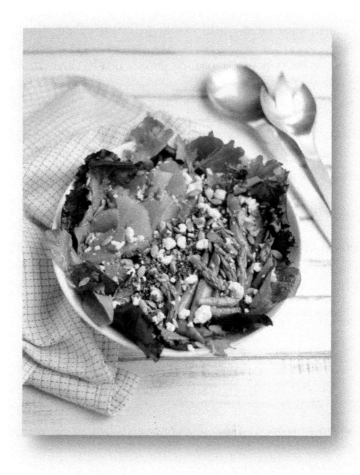

Prep Time: 10 min

Cook Time: 15 min

Serve: 2

Ingredients:

- ¼ cup minced fresh parsley

- ¼ cup slivered almonds, toasted

- 1 lb. asparagus, trimmed and cut into 1-inch lengths 1 shallot, minced

- 1 tsp. grated lemon zest plus

- 3 tbsp. juice

- 1½ cups long-grain brown rice

- 2 oz. goat cheese, crumbled (½ cup)

- 3½ tbsp. extra-virgin olive oil

- Salt and pepper

Preparation:

1. Bring 4 quarts water to boil in a Dutch oven. Put in rice and 1½ tsp. salt and cook, stirring intermittently, until rice is tender, about half an hour. Drain rice, spread onto rimmed baking sheet, and drizzle with 1 tbsp. lemon juice. Allow it to cool completely, about fifteen minutes.

2. Heat 1 tbsp. oil in 12-inch frying pan on high heat until just smoking. Put in asparagus, ¼ tsp. salt, and ¼ tsp. pepper and cook, stirring intermittently, until asparagus is browned and crisp-tender, about 4 minutes; move to plate and allow to cool slightly.

3. Beat remaining 2½ tbsp. oil, lemon zest and remaining 2 tbsp. juice, shallot, ½ tsp. salt, and ½ tsp. pepper together in a big container. Put in rice, asparagus, 2 tbsp. goat cheese, 3 tbsp. almonds, and 3 tbsp. parsley. Gently toss to combine and allow to sit for about ten minutes. Sprinkle with salt and pepper to taste.

4. Move to serving platter and drizzle with remaining 2 tbsp. goat cheese, remaining 1 tbsp. almonds, and remaining 1 tbsp. parsley. Serve.

Carrot-Almond-Bulgur Salad

Prep Time: 10 min

Cook Time: 20 min

Serve: 4

Ingredients:

- 1/8 tsp. cayenne pepper

- 1/3 cup chopped fresh cilantro

- 1/3 cup chopped fresh mint

- 1/3 cup extra-virgin olive oil

- ½ cup sliced almonds, toasted

- ½ tsp. ground cumin

- 1 cup water

- 1½ cups medium-grind bulgur, rinsed

- 3 scallions, sliced thin

- 4 carrots, peeled and shredded

- 6 tbsp. lemon juice (2 lemons)

- Salt and pepper

Preparation:

1. Mix bulgur, water, ¼ cup lemon juice, and ¼ tsp. salt in a container. Cover and sit at room temperature until grains are softened and liquid is fully absorbed, about 1½ hours.

2. Beat remaining 2 tbsp. lemon juice, oil, cumin, cayenne, and ½ tsp. salt together in a big container.

3. Put in bulgur, carrots, scallions, almonds, mint, and cilantro and gently toss to combine. Sprinkle with salt and pepper to taste. Serve.

Chickpea-Spinach Bulgur

Prep Time: 5 min

Cook Time: 20 min

Serve: 6

Ingredients:

- ¾ cup chicken or vegetable broth

- ¾ cup water

- 1 (15-oz.) can chickpeas, rinsed

- 1 cup medium-grind bulgur, rinsed

- 1 onion, chopped fine

- 1 tbsp. lemon juice

- 2 tbsp. za'atar

- 3 garlic cloves, minced

- 3 oz. (3 cups) baby spinach, chopped

- 3 tbsp. extra-virgin olive oil

- Salt and pepper

Preparation:

1. Heat 2 tbsp. oil in a big saucepan on moderate heat until it starts to shimmer. Put in onion and ½ tsp. salt and cook till they become tender, approximately five minutes. Mix in garlic and 1 tbsp. za'atar and cook until aromatic, approximately half a minute.

2. Mix in bulgur, chickpeas, broth, and water and bring to simmer. Decrease heat to low, cover, and simmer gently until bulgur is tender, 16 to 18 minutes.

3. Remove from the heat, lay clean dish towel underneath lid and let bulgur sit for about ten minutes. Put in spinach, lemon juice, remaining 1 tbsp. za'atar, and residual 1 tbsp. oil and fluff gently with fork to combine. Sprinkle with salt and pepper to taste. Serve.

Classic Baked Brown Rice

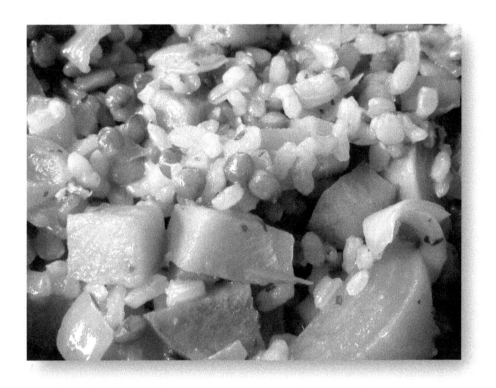

Prep Time: 10 min

Cook Time: 20 min

Serve: 6

Ingredients:

- 1½ cups long-grain brown rice, rinsed

- 2 tsp. extra-virgin olive oil

- 2 1/3 cups boiling water

- Salt and pepper

Preparation:

1. Place the oven rack in the centre of the oven and pre-heat your oven to 375°F. Mix boiling water, rice, oil, and ½ tsp. salt in 8-inch square baking dish. Cover dish tightly using double layer of aluminium foil. Bake until rice becomes soft and water is absorbed, about 1 hour. Remove the dish from oven, uncover, and gently fluff rice with fork, scraping up any rice stuck to the bottom.

2. Cover dish with clean dish towel and let rice sit for about five minutes. Uncover and let rice sit for about five minutes longer. Sprinkle with salt and pepper to taste. Serve.

Classic Italian Seafood Risotto

Prep Time: 10 min

Cook Time: 20 min

Serve: 4

Ingredients:

- 1/8 tsp. saffron threads, crumbled

- 1 (14.5-oz.) can diced tomatoes, drained

- 1 cup dry white wine

- 1 onion, chopped fine

- 1 tbsp. lemon juice

- 1 tsp. minced fresh thyme or ¼ tsp. dried

- 12 oz. large shrimp (26 to 30 per lb.), peeled and deveined, shells reserved

- 12 oz. small bay scallops

- 2 bay leaves

- 2 cups Arborio rice

- 2 cups chicken broth

- 2 tbsp. minced fresh parsley

- 2½ cups water

- 4 (8-oz.) bottles clam juice

- 5 garlic cloves, minced

- 5 tbsp. extra-virgin olive oil

- Salt and pepper

Preparation:

1. Bring shrimp shells, broth, water, clam juice, tomatoes, and bay leaves to boil in a big saucepan on moderate to high heat. Decrease the heat to a simmer and cook for 20 minutes. Strain mixture through fine-mesh strainer into big container, pressing on solids to extract as much liquid as possible; discard solids. Return broth to now-empty saucepan, cover, and keep warm on low heat.

2. Heat 2 tbsp. oil in a Dutch oven on moderate heat until it starts to shimmer. Put in onion and cook till they become tender, approximately five minutes.

3. Put in rice, garlic, thyme, and saffron and cook, stirring often, until grain edges begin to turn translucent, approximately three minutes.

4. Put in wine and cook, stirring often, until fully absorbed, approximately three minutes. Mix in 3½ cups warm broth, bring to simmer, and cook, stirring intermittently, until almost fully absorbed, about fifteen minutes.

5. Carry on cooking rice, stirring often and adding warm broth, 1 cup at a time, every few minutes as liquid is absorbed, until

rice is creamy and cooked through but still somewhat firm in center, about fifteen minutes.

6. Mix in shrimp and scallops and cook, stirring often, until opaque throughout, approximately three minutes. Remove pot from heat, cover, and allow to sit for about five minutes.

7. Adjust consistency with remaining warm broth as required (you may have broth left over). Mix in remaining 3 tbsp. oil, parsley, and lemon juice and sprinkle with salt and pepper to taste. Serve.

Classic Stovetop White Rice

Prep Time: 10 min

Cook Time: 10 min

Serve: 6

Ingredients:

- 1 tbsp. extra-virgin olive oil

- 2 cups long-grain white rice, rinsed

- 3 cups water

- long-grain rice can substitute basmati, jasmine, or Texmati rice for the long-grain rice.

- Salt and pepper

Preparation:

1. Heat oil in a big saucepan on moderate heat until it starts to shimmer. Put in rice and cook, stirring frequently, until grain edges begin to turn translucent, approximately two minutes. Put in water and 1 tsp. salt and bring to simmer.

2. Cover, decrease the heat to low, and simmer gently until rice becomes soft and water is absorbed, approximately twenty minutes. Remove from the heat, lay clean dish towel underneath lid and let rice sit for about ten minutes.

3. Gently fluff rice with fork. Sprinkle with salt and pepper to taste. Serve.

Chicken Sausage Minestrone

Ingredients:

- 4 sliced chicken sausage

- 4 tomatoes; sliced and peeled

- 2 chopped cloves

- ½ pound of diced green beans

- 2 sliced carrots

- A dubbed zucchini

- Olive oil;

- 2 tablespoons

- 1 diced sweet onion

- ½ cup of green peas; frozen

- 1 sliced celery stalk

- 2 cups of vegetable stalk

- ½ cup of marjoram; dried

- Water; 6 cups

- ½ teaspoon of oregano; dried

- ½ teaspoon of basil; dried

- Pepper and salt to taste

Preparation:

1. Get a soup pot and heat the oil, then pour in your chicken sausage and some diced onion, then cook for 5 minutes.

2. Now, add in your tomatoes, carrot, cloves, onion and celery and wait till it's cooked for another 10 minutes then add your remaining Ingredients. Add pepper and salt to taste, then cook for 20 minutes.

3. Serve and enjoy your soup when warm.

Italian Lentil soup

Ingredients:

- 2 tablespoons of sliced parsley

- Tomato paste; 2 tablespoons

- Olive Oil; 2 tablespoons

- 2 sliced cloves

- 1 cup of sliced tomatoes

- 2 celery stalks; chopped

- 2 sliced shallots

- 2 carrots; chopped

- ¼ cup of red wine

- Water; 6 cups

- A basil sprig

- A thyme sprigs

- An oregano sprig

- Green lentils; 1 cup

- 2 cups of vegetable stock

- Pepper and salt to taste

-

Preparation:

1. Get a soup pot and heat your olive oil, then pour in your chopped celery, clove, carrots and shallot, then cook for 5 minutes before adding your vegetable stock, lentils, tomatoes, wine and water.

2. Join in the herbs, then add pepper and salt to taste and then cook for 25 minutes.

3. After 25 minutes, add your sliced parsley in and serve your warm soup.

Smoked chicken sausage soup

Ingredients:

- 2 sliced chicken sausage

- 2 sliced smoked chicken sausage

- 1 can of sliced tomatoes

- 1 onion, sliced

- Water; 2 cups

- Vegetable stock; 2 cups

- 1 celery stalk; chopped

- Chopped cilantro; 2 tablespoons

- Olive Oil; 2 tablespoons

- Pepper and salt to taste

Preparation:

1. Get a soup pot and heat your olive oil, then pour in your sausage and cook for 5 minutes. After that, pour in your sliced onion, tomatoes, celery and carrots and cook for another 5 minutes.

2. Now, add your short pasta and water with pepper and salt to taste, then cook for 20 minutes. After 20 minutes, pour in your chopped parsley and cilantro then serve after cooling.

Bulgur, Kale and Cheese Mix

Prep Time: 10 min

Cook Time: 10 min

Serve: 6

Ingredients:

- 4 ounces bulgur

- 4 ounces kale, chopped

- 1 tablespoon mint, chopped

- 3 spring onions, chopped

- 1 cucumber, chopped

- A pinch of allspice, ground

- 2 tablespoons olive oil

- Zest and juice of ½ lemon

- 4 ounces feta cheese, crumbled

Preparation:

1. Put bulgur in a bowl, cover with hot water, aside for 10 minutes and fluff with a fork.

2. Heat a pan with the oil over medium heat, add the onions and the allspice and cook for 3 minutes. Add the bulgur and the rest of the ingredients, cook everything for 5-6 minutes more, divide between plates and serve.

Lemon Chicken Soup

Prep Time: 10 min

Cook Time: 20 min

Serve: 6

Ingredients:

- 10 cups chicken broth

- 3 tbsp. olive oil

- 8 cloves garlic, minced

- 1 sweet onion, sliced

- 1 large lemon, zested

- 2 boneless skinless chicken breasts

- 1 cup Israeli couscous

- 1/2 tsp. crushed red pepper

- 2 oz. crumbled feta

- 1/3 cup chopped chive

- Salt and pepper, to taste

Preparation:

1. Grab a stock pot, add the oil and place over a medium heat. Add the onion and garlic and cook for five minutes until soft. Add the broth, chicken breasts, lemon zest and crushed pepper.

2. Raise the heat, cover and bring to a boil. Reduce the heat then simmer for 5 minutes. Turn off the heat, remove the lid and remove the chicken from the pot.

3. Pop onto a place and use two forks to shred. Pop back into the pot, add the feta, chives and salt and pepper.

4. Stir well then serve and enjoy.

Tuscan Vegetable Pasta Soup

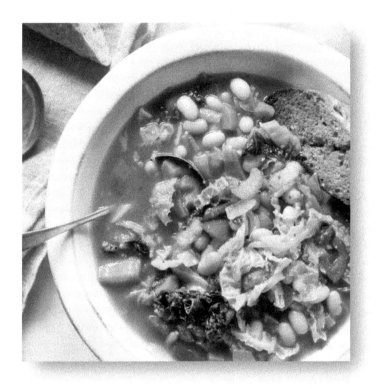

Prep Time: 10 min

Cook Time: 30 min

Serve: 6

Ingredients:

- 2 tbsp. extra virgin olive oil

- 4 cloves garlic, minced

- 1 medium yellow onion, diced

- 1/2 cup carrot, chopped

- 1/2 cup celery, chopped

- 1 medium zucchini, sliced and quartered

- 1 x 15 oz. can diced tomatoes

- 6 cups vegetable stock

- 2 tbsp. tomato paste

- 6-8 oz. whole wheat pasta

- 1 x 15 oz. can white beans

- 2 large handfuls baby spinach

- 6 basil cubes

- Salt and pepper, to taste

- Fresh chopped parsley, for garnish

Preparation:

1. Grab a stock pot, add the oil and pop over a medium heat.

2. Add the onion and garlic and cook for five minutes until soft. Throw in the carrots, celery and zucchini and cook for an extra 5 minutes, stirring occasionally.

3. Add the tomato and salt and pepper and cook for 1-2 minutes. Add the veggies broth and tomato paste, stir well then bring to the boil. Throw in the pasta, cook for 10 minutes then add the spinach, white beans, basil cubes and seasoning. Stir well then remove from the heat.

4. Divide between large bowls and serve and enjoy.

Dairy Free Zucchini Soup

Prep Time: 10 min

Cook Time: 25 min

Serve: 8

Ingredients:

- 2½ lb. zucchini

- 1 medium onion, diced

- 2 tbsp. olive oil

- 4 garlic cloves, chopped

- 4 cups chicken stock

- Sea salt and pepper, to taste

- 1/3 cup fresh basil leaves

Preparation:

1. Grab a pan, add the oil and pop over a medium heat. Add the onion, garlic and zucchini and cook for five minutes until soft. Add the stock and simmer for 15 minutes.

2. Remove from the heat, stir through the basil, add the seasoning and use an immersion blender to whizz until smooth. Serve and enjoy.

Farro Stew with Kale & Cannellini Beans

Prep Time: 10 min

Cook Time: 1 h

Serve: 4

Ingredients:

- 2 tbsp. olive oil

- 2 medium carrots, diced

- 1 medium onion, chopped

- 2 sticks celery, chopped

- 4 cloves garlic, minced

- 5 cups low-sodium vegetable broth

- 1 x 14.5 oz. can diced tomatoes

- 1 cup farro, rinsed

- 1 tsp. dried oregano

- 1 bay leaf

- Salt, to taste

- 1/2 cup parsley

- 4 cups chopped kale, thick ribs removed

- 1 x 15 oz. can cannellini beans, drained and rinsed

- 1 tbsp. fresh lemon juice

- 1/2 cup feta cheese, crumbled

Preparation:

1. Grab a stock pot, add the oil and place over a medium heat. Add the onion, carrots and celery and cook for five minutes until becoming soft.

2. Add the garlic and cook for another 30 seconds. Stir through the broth, tomatoes, farro, oregano, bay leaf, parsley and salt.

3. Cover with the lid and bring to the boil. Reduce the heat then simmer for 20 minutes. Remove the lid, add the kale and cook for a further 10-15 minutes.

4. Remove the bay leaf, add the beans, stir through the lemon juice and any additional liquid then stir well to combine. Serve and enjoy.

Italian Meatball Soup

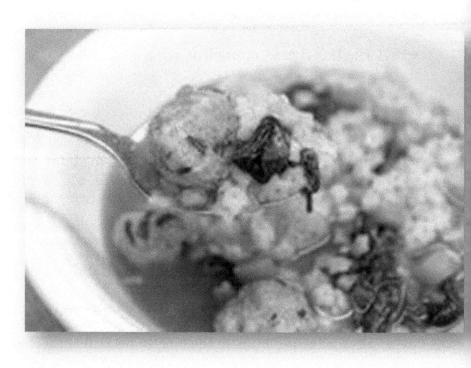

Prep Time: 10 min

Cook Time: 45 min

Serve: 6

Ingredients:

- 1/4 - 1/2 cup freshly grated parmesan cheese (optional)

- 1 free-range egg

- 1 cup breadcrumbs, optional

- 2 tbsp. fresh parsley, minced

55

- 1 tsp. dried oregano

- 1/2 tsp. sea salt

- ½ tsp. black pepper

- 3 tbsp. olive oil

- 2 quarts chicken broth or beef broth

- 3 tbsp. tomato paste

- 1 onion, diced

- 2 bay leaves

- 4-5 sprigs fresh thyme

- ½ tsp. whole black peppercorns

- Fresh parmesan cheese, grated

- 1-2 tbsp. fresh basil leaves, torn 1-2 tbsp. fresh parsley, chopped

- Salt and pepper, to taste

Preparation:

1. Place all the meatball ingredients except the oil into a medium bowl. Using your hands, mix well and form into meatballs. Place the oil into a stock pot, place over a medium heat and add the meatballs, browning on all sides.

2. Remove the meatballs from the pan. Add more oil to the pan if needed and then add the onion. Cook for five minutes until soft. Add the remaining soup ingredients, stir well then cook for 10 minutes.

3. Return the meatballs to the pan and simmer for a few minutes to warm through. Serve and enjoy.

Tuscan White Bean Soup with Sausage and Kale

Prep Time: 10 min

Cook Time: 40 min

Serve: 6

Ingredients:

- ¼ cup extra virgin olive oil

- 1 lb. hot sausage,

- 1 onion, chopped

- 1 carrot, chopped

- 1 stalk celery, chopped

- 2 cloves garlic, chopped

- ½ lb. kale, stems removed and chopped

- 4 cups chicken broth

- 1 x 28 oz. can cannelloni beans, rinsed and drained

- 1 tsp. rosemary, dried

- 1 bay leaf

- ¼ tsp. pepper

- Salt, to taste

- ½ cup shredded parmesan

Preparation:

1. Find a stock pot, pop over a medium heat and add the oil.

2. Cook the sausage until browned on all sides. Throw in the onion, carrot, celery and garlic then cook for a further five minutes. Add the kale and stir through.

3. Next add the broth, beans, rosemary and bay leaf. Stir well, bring to the boil then cover with the lid.

4. Turn down the heat then simmer for 30 minutes.

Vegetable Soup

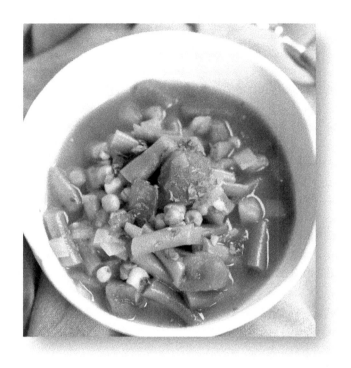

Prep Time: 10 min

Cook Time: 45 min

Serve: 4

Ingredients:

- Extra virgin olive oil, to taste

- 8 oz. sliced baby Bella mushrooms

- 2 medium-size zucchinis, sliced

- 1 bunch flat leaf parsley, chopped

- 1 red onion, chopped

- 2 garlic cloves, chopped

- 2 celery ribs, chopped

- 2 carrots, peeled, chopped

- 2 golden potatoes, peeled, diced

- 1 tsp. ground coriander

- 1/2 tsp. turmeric powder

- 1/2 tsp. sweet paprika

- 1/2 tsp. thyme Salt and pepper

- 1 x 32 oz. can whole peeled tomatoes

- 2 bay leaves

- 6 cups turkey or vegetable broth

- 1 x 15 oz. can garbanzo beans, rinsed and drained

- Juice and zest of 1 lime

- 1/3 cup toasted pine nuts, optional

Preparation:

1. Grab a large stockpot, add a tbsp. of olive oil and pop over a medium heat. Add the mushrooms and cook for five minutes, stirring often. Remove from the pan and pop to one side.

2. Add the sliced zucchini and cook for another five minutes. Remove from the pan. Add more oil and add the parsley, onions, garlic, celery, carrots and potatoes. Stir through the spices, salt and pepper.

3. Cook for five minutes until the veggies are softening. Add the tomatoes, bay leaves and broth then bring to a boil.

4. Cover and cook on medium low for 15 minutes. Remove the lid and add the garbanzo beans, mushrooms and zucchini. Heat then serve and enjoy.

Sweet Yogurt Bulgur Bowl

Prep Time: 10 min

Cook Time: 0 min

Serve: 4

Ingredients:

- 1 cup grapes, halved

- ½ cup bulgur, cooked

- ¼ cup celery stalk, chopped

- 2 oz walnuts, chopped

- ¼ cup plain yogurt

- ½ tsp. ground cinnamon

Preparation:

Mix grapes with bulgur, celery stalk, and walnut Then add plain yogurt and ground cinnamon. Stir the mixture with the help of the spoon and transfer in the serving bowls.

Spring Farro Plate

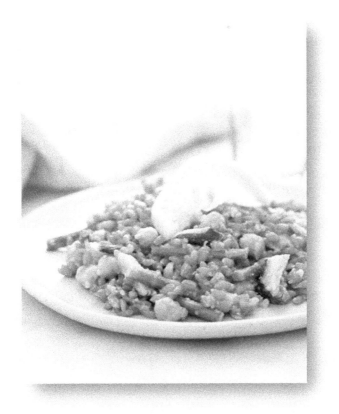

Prep Time: 15 min

Cook Time: 0 min

Serve: 6

Ingredients:

- 1 cup farro, cooked

- 2 cups baby spinach

- 2 grapefruits, roughly chopped

- 2 tbsp. balsamic vinegar

- ¼ tsp. white pepper

- 1 tbsp. olive oil

Preparation:

1. Mix baby spinach and farro in the big bowl. Then add grapefruit and shake the ingredients well.

2. Transfer the mixture in the serving plates and sprinkle with white pepper, olive oil, and balsamic vinegar.

Sorghum Taboule

Prep Time: 10 min

Cook Time: 0 min

Serve: 2

Ingredients:

- 2 oz sorghum, cooked

- 3 oz pumpkin, diced, boiled

- ½ white onion, diced 1 date, pitted, chopped

- 1 tbsp. avocado oil

- ½ tsp. liquid honey

- 2 oz Feta, crumbled

Preparation:

1. Put sorghum, pumpkin, onion, and date in the big bowl.

2. Then sprinkle the ingredients with avocado oil and liquid honey. Stir well. Transfer the cooked taboule in the serving plates and top with crumbled feta.

Spicy Green Beans Mix

Prep Time: 5 min

Cook Time: 15 min

Serve: 4

Ingredients:

- 4 teaspoons olive oil

- 1 garlic clove, minced

- ½ teaspoon hot paprika

- ¾ cup veggie stock

- 1 yellow onion, sliced

- 1 pound green beans, trimmed and halved

- ½ cup goat cheese, shredded

- 2 teaspoons balsamic vinegar

Preparation:

1. Heat a pan with the oil over medium heat, add the garlic, stir and cook for 1 minute.

2. Add the green beans and the rest of the ingredients, toss, cook everything for 15 minutes more, divide between plates and serve as a side dish.

Beans and Rice

Prep Time: 10 min

Cook Time: 55 min

Serve: 6

Ingredients:

- 1 tablespoon olive oil

- 1 yellow onion, chopped

- 2 celery stalks, chopped

- 2 garlic cloves, minced

- 2 cups brown rice

- 1 and ½ cup canned black beans, rinsed and drained

- 4 cups water

- Salt and black pepper to the taste

Preparation:

1. Heat a pan with the oil over medium heat, add the celery, garlic and the onion, stir and cook for 10 minutes.

2. Add the rest of the ingredients, stir, bring to a simmer and cook over medium heat for 45 minutes.

3. Divide between plates and serve.

Tomato and Millet Mix

Prep Time: 10 min

Cook Time: 20 min

Serve: 6

Ingredients:

- 3 tablespoons olive oil

- 1 cup millet

- 2 spring onions, chopped

- 2 tomatoes, chopped

- ½ cup cilantro, chopped

- 1 teaspoon chili paste

- 6 cups cold water

- ½ cup lemon juice

- Salt and black pepper to the taste

Preparation:

Heat a pan with the oil over medium heat, add the millet, stir and cook for 4 minutes. Add the water, salt and pepper, stir, and bring a simmer over medium heat cook for 15 minutes. Add the rest of the ingredients, toss, divide the mix between plates and serve as a side dish.

Quinoa and Greens Salad

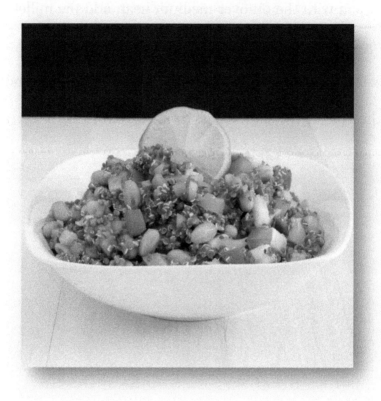

Prep Time: 10 min

Cook Time: 0 min

Serve: 4

Ingredients:

- 1 cup quinoa, cooked

- 1 medium bunch collard greens, chopped

- 4 tablespoons walnuts, chopped

- 2 tablespoons balsamic vinegar

- 4 tablespoons tahini paste

- 4 tablespoons cold water

- A pinch of salt and black pepper

- 1 tablespoon olive oil

Preparation:

In a bowl, mix the tahini with the water and vinegar and whisk.

In a bowl, mix the quinoa with the rest of the ingredients and the tahini dressing, toss, divide the mix between plates and serve as a side dish.

Veggies and Avocado Dressing

Prep Time: 10 min

Cook Time: 0 min

Serve: 4

Ingredients:

- 3 tablespoons pepitas, roasted

- 3 cups water

- 2 tablespoons cilantro, chopped

- 4 tablespoons parsley, chopped

- 1 and ½ cups corn

- 1 cup radish, sliced

- 2 avocados, peeled, pitted and chopped

- 2 mangos, peeled and chopped

- 3 tablespoons olive oil

- 4 tablespoons Greek yogurt

- 1 teaspoon balsamic vinegar

- 2 tablespoons lime juice

- Salt and black pepper to the taste

Preparation:

In your blender, mix the olive oil with avocados, salt, pepper, lime juice, the yogurt and the vinegar and pulse. In a bowl, mix the pepitas with the cilantro, parsley and the rest of the ingredients, and toss. Add the avocado dressing, toss, divide the mix between plates and serve as a side dish.

Sugar-coated Pecans

Prep Time: 15 min

Cook Time: 1 h

Serve: 12

Ingredients:

- 1 egg white

- 1 tablespoon water

- 1 pound pecan halves

- 1 cup white sugar

- 3/4 teaspoon salt

- 1/2 teaspoon ground cinnamon

Preparation:

1. Preheat the oven to 120 ° C (250 ° F). Grease a baking tray. In a bowl, whisk the egg whites and water until frothy. 2. Combine the sugar, salt, and cinnamon in another bowl.

3. Add the pecans to the egg whites and stir to cover the nuts. Remove the nuts and mix them with the sugar until well covered. Spread the nuts on the prepared baking sheet.

4. Bake for 1 hour at 250 ° F (120 ° C). Stir every 15 minutes.

Southwestern Egg Rolls

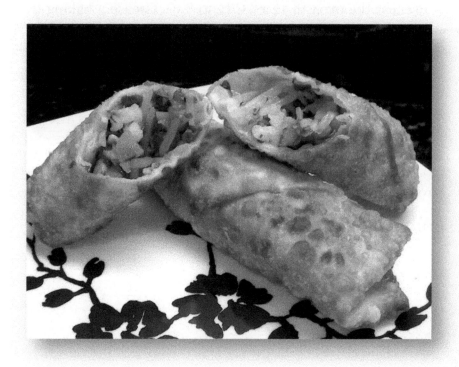

Prep Time: 20 min

Cook Time: 20 min

Serve: 5

Ingredients:

- 2 tablespoons vegetable oil

- 1/2 chicken fillet, skinless

- 2 tablespoons chopped green onion

- 2 tablespoons chopped red pepper

- 1/3 cup frozen corn kernels

- 1/4 cup black beans, rinsed and drained

- 2 tablespoons chopped frozen spinach, thawed and drained 2 tablespoons diced jalapeño peppers

- 1/2 tablespoon chopped fresh parsley

- 1/2 c. ground cumin

- 1/2 teaspoon chili powder

- 1/3 teaspoon salt

- 1 pinch of ground cayenne pepper

- 3/4 cup of grated Monterey Jack cheese

- 5 flour tortillas (6 inches)

- 1 liter of oil for frying

Preparation:

1. Rub 1 tablespoon of vegetable oil on the chicken fillet. Cook the chicken in a medium-sized saucepan over medium heat for about 5 minutes per side until the meat is no longer pink and the juice is clear. Remove from heat and set aside.

2. Heat 1 tablespoon of remaining vegetable oil in a medium-sized saucepan over medium heat. Stir in the green onion and red pepper. Boil and stir for 5 minutes, until soft.

3. Cut the diced chicken and mix in the pan with the onion and red pepper. Mix corn, black beans, spinach, jalapeño pepper, parsley, cumin, chili powder, salt, and cayenne pepper. Boil and stir for 5 minutes, until everything is well mixed and soft. Remove from heat and stir in Monterey Jack cheese until it melts.

4. Wrap the tortillas with a clean, slightly damp cloth — microwave at maximum power, about 1 minute, or until it is hot and malleable. Pour equal amounts of the mixture into each tortilla. Fold the ends of the tortillas and wrap the mixture well. Safe with toothpicks. Arrange in a medium-sized dish, cover with plastic, and place in the freezer.

5. Freeze for at least 4 hours. Heat the oil in a deep frying pan to 190° C for frying. Bake frozen stuffed tortillas for 10 minutes or until golden brown. Drain on paper towels before serving.

Roasted Vegetable soup

Ingredients:

- Vegetable stock; 2 cups

- 2 sliced red bell pepper

- 4 tomatoes; diced

- 2 cups of water

- A sprig of rosemary

- Olive oil; 3 tablespoons

- 1 sliced carrot

- 2 red onions; cut in halves

- 4 cloves

- Pepper and salt to taste

- A small butternut; crushed, peeled and diced

Preparation:

1. Get a baking tray and add your carrot, cloves, tomatoes, red onions, parsnip, bell pepper, rosemary and crushed butternut. Add pepper and salt to taste then drizzle with oil.

2. Now, preheat your oven to 350F, then cook for 25-30 minutes till it turns golden brown. Move your vegetable into a soup pot and add in the stock and some water then cook for another 10 minutes.

3. After 10 minutes, remove the rosemary then grind with an immersion blender. Enjoy your soup when warm.

Mediterranean Chicken Soup

Ingredients:

- 2 sliced cloves

- 2 peeled and sliced tomatoes

- A bay leaf

- 1 juiced lemon

- 1 sweet onion; diced

- 1 cubed zucchini

- Water; 4 cups

- ½ teaspoon of capers; sliced

- ½ teaspoon of oregano; dried

- Dried basil; 1 teaspoon

- ½ cup of orzo

- Chicken stock; 2 cups

- 1 pound of chicken drumsticks

- 1 chopped and cored green bell pepper

- 1 chopped and cored red bell pepper

- Pepper and salt to taste

-

Preparation:

1. Get a soup pot and add your vegetable, stock, herbs, chicken, bay leaf and water together, then add pepper and salt to taste and cook on low heat for 25 minutes.

2. Now add your lemon juice and cook again for 5 minutes.

3. Serve and enjoy your warm soup.

Mediterranean Bean and Sausage soup

Ingredients:

- Olive oil; 2 tablespoons

- A can of drained black beans

- Juiced tomato; 1 cup

- 4 cups of water

- 1 pound of sliced chicken sausage

- 2 cups of chicken stalk

- 1 chopped celery stalk

- 2 sliced cloves

- 1 can of drained kidney beans

- 1 sliced carrot

- 2 peeled and sliced tomatoes

- A rosemary sprig

- 1 bay leaf

- A sweet onion; diced

- Pepper and salt to taste

-

Preparation:

1. Get a soup pot and heat your olive oil, then pour in your sausage and cook for 5 minutes. Now, add all other Ingredients.

2. Add pepper and salt to taste and cook for 25 minutes.

3. Serve and enjoy when cooled

Spicy Avocado soup

Ingredients:

- 2 tablespoons of olive oil
- 1 cored and sliced red pepper
- 2 peeled and sliced avocado
- Water; 4 cups
- A sprig of thyme
- Baby spinach; 2 cups
- A sprig of oregano
- 2 sliced cloves
- 1 sliced celery stalk
- 2 cups of vegetable stock
- 1 sliced shallot
- ¼ cup of sliced cilantro
- 1 chopped jelapeno
- Pepper and salt to taste

Preparation:

1. Get a soup pot and heat your olive oil, then pour in your sliced celery, clove, oregano, shallot, red pepper and thyme.

2.. Now, pour in your chopped jelapeno, stock and water then add pepper and salt to taste and cook on low heat for 10 minutes. Add your spinach and cook for 10 minutes again. Now, pour the soup into serving bowls and add your avocado and cilantro slice on top. Serve and enjoy.

Smoked Ham and Split Pea soup

Ingredients:

- Water; 6 cups

- ½ cup of split pea

- 1 sliced jelapeno pepper

- 4 Oz of diced smoked ham

- 2 carrots; chopped

- 2 tomatoes; peeled and sliced

- 1 diced sweet onion

- 1 sliced parsnip

- 2 cups of vegetable stock

- 1 juiced lemon

- Olive oil; 2 tablespoons

- 2 carrots; sliced

- 2 cloves; sliced

- 2 red bell pepper; cored and sliced

- Creme fraiche to serve

Preparation:

1. Get a soup pot and heat your olive oil, then pour in your ham and cook for 5 minutes, then pour the rest of your ingredients. Add pepper and salt to taste, then cook for 30 minutes with low heat.

2. Serve your warm soup topped with creme fraiche and enjoy.

Annie's Salsa Chips with Fruit & Cinnamon

Prep Time: 15 min

Cook Time: 15 min

Serve: 10

Ingredients:

- 2 Golden Delicious apples - peeled, seeded and diced

- 8 grams of raspberry

- 2 kiwis, peeled and diced

- 1 pound of strawberries

- 2 tablespoons of white sugar 1 tablespoon of brown sugar

- 3 tablespoons canned fruit Flour cooking aerosol

- Flour tortillas

- 2 tablespoons cinnamon sugar

Preparation:

1. Combine kiwi, Golden Delicious apples, raspberries, strawberries, white sugar, brown sugar, and canned fruit in a large bowl. Cover and put in the fridge for at least 15 minutes. Preheat the oven to 175 ° C (350 ° F).

2. Cover one side of each flour tortilla with a cooking spray. 3. Cut into segments and place them in one layer on a large baking sheet. Sprinkle the quarters with the desired amount of cinnamon sugar.

4. Spray again with cooking spray. Bake in the preheated oven for 8 to 10 minutes. Repeat this with the other tortilla quarters. Cool for approximately 15 minutes. Serve with a mixture of fresh fruit.

Boneless Buffalo Wings

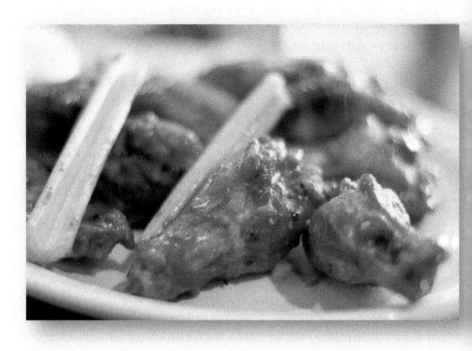

Prep Time: 10 min

Cook Time: 15 min

Serve: 3

Ingredients:

- Frying oil

- 1 cup unbleached flour

- 2 teaspoons of salt

- 1/2 teaspoon ground black pepper

- 1/2 teaspoon cayenne pepper

- 1/4 teaspoon garlic powder

- 1/2 teaspoon bell pepper

- 1 egg

- 1 cup of milk

- 3 boneless chicken fillets, skinless, cut into 1/2 inch strips 1/4 cup hot pepper sauce

- 1 tablespoon butter

Preparation:

1. Heat the oil in a frying pan or large saucepan.

2. Mix the flour, salt, black pepper, cayenne pepper, garlic powder, and bell pepper in a large bowl. Beat the egg and milk in a small bowl. Dip each piece of chicken in the egg mixture and then roll it into the flour mixture. Repeat the process so that each piece of chicken is doubled. Cool the breaded chicken for 20 minutes.

3. Fry chicken in hot oil, in batches. Cook until the outside is well browned and the juice is clear, 5 to 6 minutes per batch.

4. Mix the hot sauce and butter in a small bowl. Heat the sauce in the microwave on high to melt, 20 to 30 seconds. Pour the sauce over the cooked chicken; mix well.

Jalapeño Popper Spread

Prep Time: 10 min

Cook Time: 3 min

Serve: 32

Ingredients:

- 2 packets of cream cheese, softened

- 1 cup mayonnaise

- 1 (4-gram) can chopped green peppers, drained

- 2 grams diced jalapeño peppers, canned, drained

- 1 cup grated Parmesan cheese

-

Preparation:

1. In a large bowl, mix cream cheese and mayonnaise until smooth. Stir the bell peppers and jalapeño peppers.

2. Pour the mixture into a microwave oven and sprinkle with Parmesan cheese. Microwave on maximum power, about 3 minutes.

Brown Sugar Smokies

Prep Time: 10 min

Cook Time: 10 min

Serve: 12

Ingredients:

- 1 pound bacon

- 1 (16 ounces) package little smoky sausages

- 1 cup brown sugar, or to taste

Preparation:

1. Preheat the oven to 175 ° C (350 ° F).

2. Cut the bacon in three and wrap each strip around a little sausage. Place sausages wrapped on wooden skewers, several to one place the kebabs on a baking sheet and sprinkle generously with brown sugar. Bake until the bacon is crispy, and the brown sugar has melted.

Pita Chips

Prep Time: 10 min

Cook Time: 8 min

Servings: 24

Ingredients:

- 12 slices of pita bread

- 1/2 cup of olive oil

- 1/2 teaspoon ground black pepper

- 1 teaspoon garlic salt

- 1/2 teaspoon dried basil

- 1 teaspoon dried chervil

Preparation:

1. Preheat the oven to 200 degrees C (400 degrees F).

2. Cut each pita bread into 8 triangles. Place the triangles on the baking sheet. Combine oil, pepper, salt, basil, and chervil in a small bowl.

3. Brush each triangle with the oil mixture. Bake in the preheated oven for about 7 minutes or until light brown and crispy.

Hot Spinach, Artichoke & Chili Dip

Prep Time: 10 min

Cook Time: 30 min

Serve: 10

Ingredients:

- 2 (8 oz.) packages of cream cheese, softened

- 1/2 cup of mayonnaise

- 1 can (4.5 oz.) chopped green pepper, drained

- 1 cup of freshly grated Parmesan cheese

- 1 jar (12 oz.) marinated artichoke hearts, drained and chopped

- 1/4 cup canned chopped jalapeño peppers, drained

- 1 can of chopped spinach frozen, thawed and drained

Preparation:

1. Preheat the oven to 175 ° C (350 ° F). Mix the cream cheese and mayonnaise in a bowl.

2. Stir the green peppers, parmesan cheese, artichokes, peppers, and spinach. Pour the mixture into a baking dish.

3. Bake in the preheated oven until light brown, about 30 minutes.

Mediterranean Beef Toss Spaghetti

Total Time: 25 min

Serve: 4

Ingredients:

- Lean ground beef - 1 2 pound

- Divided salt - 3 4 teaspoon

- Pepper - 1 4 teaspoon

- Medium red onion, sliced - 1

- Medium green pepper, cut into 1-inch pieces - 1

- Diced tomatoes, undrained - 1 can (28 ounces)

- Red wine vinegar - 1 teaspoon

- Dried basil - 1 teaspoon

- Dried thyme - 1 teaspoon

- 2 medium zucchinis, sliced

- 3 teaspoons of olive oil, divided

- 4 garlic cloves, minced

- Hot cooked spaghetti (optional)

Preparation:

1. Cook the beef, garlic, 1 4 teaspoon salt and pepper in 1 teaspoon oil in a nonstick pan over medium heat until meat is no longer pink Drain the pan after the meat has cooked.

2. Empty the pan into a bowl and keep warm. Sauté the onion in oil for 2 minutes using the same pan. Pour zucchini and green pepper into the pan, and stir continuously for 4-6 minutes or until vegetables are crispy soft.

3. Add tomatoes, vinegar, basil, thyme and remaining salt (½ teaspoon) and mix properly.

4. Add beef mixture and heat properly. Serve with spaghetti.

Herb-Crusted Mediterranean Pork Tenderloin

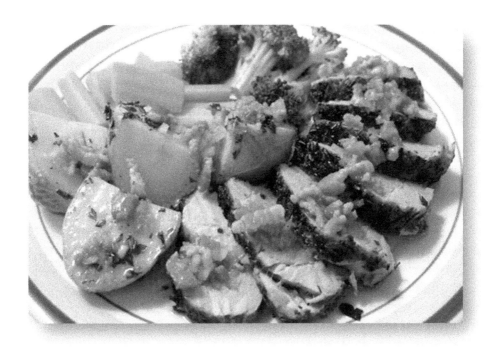

Total Time: 35 min

Serve: 3

Ingredients:

- Pork tenderloin – 3 4 pound

- Olive oil - 3 4 tablespoon

- Dried oregano – 1½ teaspoons

- Lemon pepper - 9 16 teaspoon

- Olive tapenade (refrigerated mixed) – 2¼ tablespoons

- Feta cheese (finely crumbled, about 3 tablespoons) - 3 4 ounce

Preparation:

1. Put pork on a large plastic wrapper. Apply oil over the tenderloin; sprinkle oregano and lemon pepper all over the surface. Tightly wind the plastic wrapper around the meat; leave in the freezer for 2 hours or overnight.

2. Start a medium heat fire in the grill. Remove meat from plastic wrapper and make a vertical cut through the middle. Do not cut completely through to the opposite side.

3. Open both halves of the meat and apply a generous amount of olive tapénade on one half — Scatter cheese all over the surface. Fold the other half to form the natural shape of tenderloin. Bind tightly with thin cord set 1½ to 2-inches apart.

4. Place the tenderloin over direct heat from the grill for 20 minutes, or the internal temperature reaches 145° F. Remember to switch the sides halfway into the grilling.

5. Move the tenderloin to the cutting board. Cover gently with foil and leave it for 5-10 minutes.

6. Remove the cord and cut into smaller pieces about 1 4-inch-thick. Ready to serve.

Lightning Source UK Ltd.
Milton Keynes UK
UKHW020640090421
381714UK00011B/320

9 781801 902830